Cucumber Fruit Guide for Beginners

Understanding the Varieties of Cucumber

By

Torin Brigham

Table of Contents

CHAPTER 1

Introduction to Cucumber Fruit

Cucumbers, scientifically known as Cucumis sativus, are one of the most widely cultivated and consumed fruits in the world. Despite being commonly mistaken for vegetables due to their culinary uses, cucumbers are botanically classified as fruits. This intriguing botanical classification arises from the fact that cucumbers develop from the flower of the cucumber plant and contain seeds within their fleshy structure, two defining characteristics of fruits.

1.1 Definition and Characteristics

The cucumber fruit typically exhibits an elongated cylindrical shape, although variations in size, shape, color, and texture exist across different cultivars. They belong to the Cucurbitaceae family, which encompasses various gourd species, including pumpkins, squash, and melons. Cucumbers are characterized by their crisp and juicy flesh, often encased in a thin, smooth skin. However, some varieties may feature ridged or bumpy exteriors.

One of the defining features of cucumbers is their high-water content, which contributes to their refreshing and hydrating properties. This attribute makes cucumbers a popular choice for salads, snacks, and beverages, particularly in hot climates where their cooling effect is especially appreciated.

cucumbers are renowned for their versatility in culinary applications. They can be consumed raw, sliced, diced, or grated, adding a crisp texture and mild flavor to a wide array of dishes. From salads and sandwiches to pickles and gazpachos, cucumbers play a prominent role in cuisines around the world, contributing both taste and nutritional value.

Beyond their culinary appeal, cucumbers boast several nutritional benefits. They are low in calories and fat while providing essential vitamins, minerals, and antioxidants. Cucumbers are particularly rich in vitamin K, vitamin C, potassium, and various phytonutrients, all of which contribute to their potential health-promoting properties.

cucumbers are relatively easy to cultivate, making them accessible to home gardeners and commercial growers alike. They thrive in temperate climates with ample sunlight and well-drained soil, although certain varieties have been adapted to grow in diverse environments.

cucumbers are botanically classified as fruits and are prized for their crisp texture, high water content, and culinary versatility. Whether eaten fresh, pickled, or incorporated into dishes, cucumbers are a ubiquitous and beloved ingredient in cuisines worldwide. Their nutritional profile and ease of cultivation further contribute to their widespread popularity, making them a staple in households and markets across the globe.

1.2 Botanical Classification

Botanically, cucumbers belong to the Cucurbitaceae family, a diverse group of flowering plants commonly referred to as the gourd family. This family encompasses a wide range of species, including cucumbers, pumpkins, squash, melons, and gourds. Within the Cucurbitaceae family, cucumbers are classified under the genus Cucumis and species sativus, giving them the scientific name Cucumis sativus.

Cucumbers are further classified taxonomically according to their botanical characteristics. They are dicotyledonous plants, meaning they produce seedlings with two embryonic leaves upon germination. Additionally, cucumbers are angiosperms, which are flowering plants that produce seeds enclosed within a fruit.

One of the distinguishing features of cucumbers is their vine-like growth habit.

Cucumber plants are sprawling vines that tend to trail along the ground or climb vertical supports using tendrils. This growth pattern is characteristic of many members of the Cucurbitaceae family, allowing them to efficiently utilize available space and resources in their natural habitats.

The cucumber fruit itself develops from the female flowers of the cucumber plant. Cucumber flowers are typically unisexual, meaning they contain either male or female reproductive organs. Female flowers, which bear the potential to develop into fruits, feature a miniature cucumber-like structure at the base of the flower known as an ovary. Once fertilized by pollen from male flowers, the ovary develops into the familiar elongated fruit that we recognize as a cucumber.

Cucumber fruits exhibit a wide range of diversity in terms of size, shape, color, and texture, reflecting the genetic variability within the species. While the classic image of a cucumber is a long, straight, green fruit with smooth skin, there are numerous cultivars that deviate from this archetype.

Varieties of cucumbers may differ in length, ranging from short pickling cucumbers to long English or slicing cucumbers. Some cucumbers may have ridged or bumpy exteriors, while others may be pale yellow or even white in color.

Cucumbers are classified taxonomically as members of the Cucurbitaceae family, genus Cucumis, and species sativus. They are dicotyledonous, angiospermous plants with vine-like growth habits. The cucumber fruit develops from the female flowers of the cucumber plant and exhibits considerable diversity in size, shape, color, and texture among different cultivars.

1.3 Historical Significance

Cucumbers have a rich history that spans thousands of years, with evidence of their cultivation and consumption dating back to ancient times. Throughout history, cucumbers have held various cultural, culinary, and medicinal significance in different civilizations around the world.

One of the earliest known origins of cucumber cultivation can be traced to the region encompassing present-day India and Nepal, where wild cucumbers were domesticated as early as 3000 BCE. From there, cucumbers spread to other parts of Asia, including China and Persia (modern-day Iran), where they became integral components of regional cuisines.

In ancient civilizations such as Egypt, cucumbers held significant cultural and religious symbolism. Archaeological findings suggest that cucumbers were cultivated along the Nile River as early as 2500 BCE, and they were depicted in Egyptian hieroglyphics and tomb paintings. Cucumbers were associated with fertility and were offered to the gods in religious rituals. Additionally, cucumbers were prized for their refreshing and hydrating properties in the arid climate of ancient Egypt.

The ancient Greeks and Romans also embraced cucumbers both for their culinary appeal and medicinal properties. Cucumbers were cultivated in ancient Greece and were mentioned in the works of prominent figures such as Theophrastus, a Greek philosopher and botanist. The Romans further popularized cucumbers throughout their empire, incorporating them into various dishes and preserving them through pickling techniques.

In medieval Europe, cucumbers gained prominence as a cultivated crop, particularly among monastic communities and nobility. Cucumbers were grown in gardens for culinary purposes and were valued for their cooling properties during the summer months. However, cucumbers were not universally embraced in Europe during this period, with some individuals expressing skepticism about their nutritional value and potential health effects.

During the Age of Exploration in the 15th and 16th centuries, European explorers and traders introduced cucumbers to the Americas and other parts of the world. Cucumbers quickly became integrated into local cuisines, with indigenous populations adopting them into traditional dishes.

In more recent history, cucumbers have remained a staple food item in many cultures, appreciated for their versatility, nutritional value, and refreshing taste. Today, cucumbers are cultivated on a global scale, with diverse varieties available year-round in markets worldwide.

Cucumbers have a long and storied history that spans multiple civilizations and time periods. From their origins in ancient Asia to their widespread cultivation and consumption in modern times, cucumbers have played significant roles in culinary traditions, cultural practices, and agricultural practices around the world.

CHAPTER 2

Cultivation of Cucumber

2.1 Growing Conditions

Cucumbers are relatively easy to cultivate, but they require specific growing conditions to thrive and produce abundant yields. Understanding and providing these optimal conditions is essential for successful cucumber cultivation. Here are the key factors to consider when growing cucumbers:

1. **Climate:**

   - Cucumbers are warm-season crops that require a long, frost-free growing season to reach maturity. They thrive in temperatures between 70°F and 95°F (21°C to 35°C).

   - Avoid planting cucumbers too early in the spring when the soil is still cold, as this can stunt their growth and increase susceptibility to diseases.

- Provide adequate protection or support for cucumber plants during periods of extreme heat, as excessive heat can stress the plants and reduce fruit quality.

2. **Sunlight:**

- Cucumbers require full sun exposure for optimal growth and fruit development. Aim for at least 6 to 8 hours of direct sunlight per day.

- Ensure that cucumber plants are not shaded by taller crops or structures, as this can hinder their growth and productivity.

3. **Soil:**

- Choose a well-drained, fertile soil with a pH level between

6.0 and 7.0. Sandy loam or loamy soils are ideal for cucumbers.

- Incorporate organic matter, such as compost or aged manure, into the soil before planting to improve its structure, fertility, and moisture retention.

- Avoid compacted or waterlogged soils, as they can inhibit root development and lead to poor growth.

4. **Watering:**

- Cucumbers have shallow root systems and require consistent moisture throughout the growing season. Keep the soil evenly moist, but not waterlogged, to prevent issues such as blossom end rot and fruit splitting.

- Provide regular irrigation, especially during dry periods and hot weather. Mulching around the base of the plants can help retain soil moisture and suppress weed growth.

5. **Spacing and Support:**

    - Plant cucumber seeds or seedlings in rows or hills with adequate spacing to promote air circulation and minimize competition for nutrients.

    - Space rows approximately 3 to 4 feet apart, with individual plants spaced 12 to 24 inches apart within the rows, depending on the cucumber variety.

    - Consider providing support for vining cucumber varieties by installing trellises, cages, or stakes. Vertical growing systems can help maximize space and reduce disease pressure by keeping fruits off the ground.

6. **Fertilization:**

- Incorporate a balanced fertilizer into the soil before planting, following recommendations based on soil test results or general guidelines for vegetable crops.

- Side-dress cucumber plants with additional fertilizer throughout the growing season to support vigorous growth and fruit production. Avoid excessive nitrogen, as it can promote lush foliage at the expense of fruit development.

Ensuring that cucumbers are grown in optimal conditions with proper care and management, growers can maximize their yields and produce high-quality fruits for fresh consumption or processing. Monitoring for pests, diseases, and environmental stressors is also crucial for maintaining healthy cucumber plants throughout the growing season.

2.2 Varieties of Cucumbers

Cucumbers come in a wide range of varieties, each with its own unique characteristics in terms of size, shape, color, flavor, and texture. The choice of cucumber variety depends on factors such as intended use (fresh consumption, pickling, or processing), growing conditions, and personal preferences. Here are some common types of cucumbers:

1. **Slicing Cucumbers:**

    - English or European cucumbers: Also known as "seedless" or "burpless" cucumbers, these varieties typically have thin, tender skins and mild, non-bitter flesh. They are longer and slimmer than traditional cucumbers, with a smoother appearance.

- American slicing cucumbers: These cucumbers are more cylindrical in shape with slightly thicker skins. They are commonly found in supermarkets and farmers' markets and are ideal for slicing into salads, sandwiches, and snacks.

2. **Pickling Cucumbers:**

- Kirby cucumbers: Named after James E. Kirby, a farmer who popularized their cultivation in the late 19th century, Kirby cucumbers are small, firm, and crunchy. They have bumpy exteriors and are well-suited for pickling due to their ability to retain crispness and flavor.

- Persian or Lebanese cucumbers: These cucumbers are shorter and stubbier than English cucumbers but longer than gherkins. They are often used for both fresh consumption and pickling, as they have thin skins and a crisp texture.

3. **Gherkin Cucumbers:**

   - Gherkins, also known as cornichons, are small, tart cucumbers commonly used for pickling. They are harvested when immature, typically measuring 1 to 3 inches in length. Gherkins are prized for their crunchy texture and tangy flavor, making them popular for use in relishes, chutneys, and condiments.

4. **Specialty Cucumbers:**

- Lemon cucumbers: These heirloom cucumbers are round or oval in shape and yellow in color, resembling small lemons. They have a mild, slightly sweet flavor and are often eaten fresh in salads or sliced for garnishes.

- Armenian cucumbers: Also known as snake cucumbers or serpentine cucumbers, Armenian cucumbers are long and slender with ribbed skins. They have a mild, crisp texture and are commonly used in Middle Eastern and Mediterranean cuisines.

5. **Hybrid and Novelty Varieties:**

- Seed companies and breeders continually develop new hybrid cucumber varieties with improved disease resistance, yield potential, and culinary qualities. These hybrids may offer unique features such as uniformity in size and shape, extended shelf life, or enhanced flavor profiles.

When selecting cucumber varieties for cultivation, it's essential to consider factors such as disease resistance, climate suitability, and intended market preferences. Additionally, home gardeners may prioritize characteristics such as compact growth habits or container-friendly varieties for small-space gardening. By exploring the diverse range of cucumber varieties available, growers can discover options that meet their specific needs and preferences, whether for fresh consumption, pickling, or culinary experimentation.

2.3 Planting and Maintenance

Successfully growing cucumbers requires attention to detail during both the planting and maintenance phases. Proper planting techniques, adequate care, and timely maintenance contribute to healthy plant development, vigorous growth, and abundant fruit production. Here's a comprehensive guide to planting and maintaining cucumber plants:

1. **Planting Time:**

   - Plant cucumbers outdoors after the last frost date in your region when soil temperatures have warmed to at least 60°F (15°C). In cooler climates, start seeds indoors 2-4 weeks before transplanting to ensure an early start.

   - Cucumbers are warm-season crops, so they require a long, frost-free growing season to reach maturity. Ensure that weather conditions are favorable for consistent growth and development.

2. **Site Selection:**

- Choose a planting site with full sun exposure (at least 6-8 hours of direct sunlight per day) and well-drained soil. Avoid low-lying areas that are prone to waterlogging, as excessive moisture can lead to root rot and other fungal diseases.

- Consider planting cucumbers near a trellis, fence, or other support structure to maximize space and encourage upward growth. Vertical gardening techniques can help conserve space and promote better air circulation around the plants.

3. **Soil Preparation:**

- Prepare the soil by loosening it to a depth of 6-8 inches and incorporating organic matter such as compost, aged manure, or peat moss to improve soil fertility and structure.

- Conduct a soil test to determine pH levels and nutrient deficiencies, and amend the soil accordingly to ensure optimal growing conditions for cucumber plants.

4. **Planting Seeds or Transplants:**

- Plant cucumber seeds directly in the garden or start them indoors in biodegradable pots filled with seed-starting mix. Sow seeds 1 inch deep and space them 6-12 inches apart in rows or hills.

- If transplanting seedlings, handle them carefully to avoid damaging the delicate roots. Plant seedlings at the same depth as they were growing in their containers, spacing them according to the recommended spacing for the chosen cucumber variety.

5. **Watering:**

- Keep the soil consistently moist but not waterlogged, especially during the germination and flowering stages. Water cucumbers deeply at the base of the plants to encourage strong root development.

- Avoid overhead watering, as wet foliage can increase the risk of foliar diseases such as powdery mildew. Use drip irrigation or soaker hoses to deliver water directly to the root zone.

6. **Fertilization:**

- Apply a balanced fertilizer or organic fertilizer at planting time to provide essential nutrients for healthy plant growth. Side-dress cucumber plants with additional fertilizer every 3-4 weeks throughout the growing season to support vigorous growth and fruit production.

- Monitor plant health and adjust fertilization practices based on soil test results, plant nutrient deficiencies, and growth rates.

7. **Weed Control:**

- Keep the area around cucumber plants free of weeds, as competition for nutrients, water, and sunlight can inhibit their growth and productivity. Mulching with organic materials such as straw, shredded leaves, or grass clippings can help suppress weeds and conserve soil moisture.

8. **Pest and Disease Management:**

- Monitor cucumber plants regularly for signs of pests such as aphids, cucumber beetles, and spider mites, as well as common diseases like powdery mildew, downy mildew, and bacterial wilt.

- Practice integrated pest management (IPM) strategies, including cultural controls, biological controls, and selective pesticide applications, to minimize pest and disease damage while minimizing environmental impact.

9. **Pruning and Training:**

- Train vining cucumber varieties to climb trellises, stakes, or other support structures to conserve space and promote better air circulation around the plants.

- Remove excess foliage and lateral branches to improve light penetration and airflow within the canopy, reducing

the risk of fungal diseases
and improving fruit quality.

10. Harvesting:

- Harvest cucumbers when
  they reach the desired size
  and color for their variety.
  Most slicing cucumbers are
  best harvested when they are
  6-8 inches long, while
  pickling cucumbers are
  typically harvested at 2-4
  inches in length.

- Use sharp garden shears or a
  knife to cut cucumbers from
  the vine, taking care not to
  damage the stems or adjacent
  fruits. Harvest cucumbers
  regularly to encourage
  continued fruit production
  throughout the growing
  season.

These planting and maintenance guidelines,
growers can optimize the growth and
productivity of cucumber plants, resulting in

a bountiful harvest of fresh, flavorful fruits for culinary enjoyment. Regular monitoring, proper care, and timely interventions are essential for managing potential challenges such as pests, diseases, and environmental stressors, ensuring successful cucumber cultivation from planting to harvest.

CHAPTER 3

Nutritional Value and Health Benefits

3.1 Macronutrients and Micronutrients

Cucumbers are not only delicious and refreshing but also pack a nutritional punch, offering a variety of essential macronutrients and micronutrients that contribute to overall health and well-being. Here's an overview of the nutritional composition of cucumbers:

Macronutrients:

1. **Water:**

   - Cucumbers are composed primarily of water, with a high water content ranging from 95% to 96% of their total weight. This makes cucumbers an excellent choice for hydration, especially during hot weather or after physical activity.

2. **Carbohydrates:**

- Cucumbers are low in carbohydrates, with approximately 3 to 4 grams of carbohydrates per 100 grams serving. The majority of these carbohydrates come from dietary fiber, which contributes to digestive health and helps regulate blood sugar levels.

3. **Protein:**

- While cucumbers are not a significant source of protein, they do contain small amounts, with approximately 0.7 to 1 gram of protein per 100 grams serving. Protein is essential for muscle growth, repair, and overall cellular function.

4. **Fats:**

- Cucumbers are virtually fat-free, containing negligible amounts of fat. This makes them an excellent choice for individuals following low-fat diets or seeking to reduce their overall fat intake.

Micronutrients:

1. **Vitamins:**

- Vitamin K: Cucumbers are a good source of vitamin K, with approximately 16 to 20 micrograms per 100 grams serving. Vitamin K plays a crucial role in blood clotting, bone health, and cardiovascular function.

- Vitamin C: Cucumbers contain moderate levels of vitamin C, with approximately 3 to 4 milligrams per 100 grams serving. Vitamin C is an

antioxidant that supports
immune function, collagen
synthesis, and wound
healing.

- Vitamin A: Cucumbers
  provide small amounts of
  vitamin A in the form of
  beta-carotene, with
  approximately 100 to 150
  international units (IU) per
  100 grams serving. Vitamin
  A is important for vision,
  skin health, and immune
  function.

- B Vitamins: Cucumbers
  contain trace amounts of
  various B vitamins, including
  B1 (thiamine), B2
  (riboflavin), B3 (niacin), B5
  (pantothenic acid), B6
  (pyridoxine), and B9 (folate).
  These vitamins play essential
  roles in energy metabolism,
  nerve function, and red blood
  cell production.

2. **Minerals:**

- Potassium: Cucumbers are a good source of potassium, with approximately 147 to 160 milligrams per 100 grams serving. Potassium is an electrolyte that helps regulate fluid balance, nerve function, and muscle contractions.

- Magnesium: Cucumbers provide small amounts of magnesium, with approximately 13 to 15 milligrams per 100 grams serving. Magnesium is involved in over 300 biochemical reactions in the body, including energy metabolism, muscle function, and bone health.

- Other Minerals: Cucumbers also contain trace amounts of other minerals such as calcium, phosphorus, zinc, and manganese, which are essential for various physiological processes in the body.

cucumbers are a nutritious addition to a balanced diet, offering a combination of essential macronutrients and micronutrients that support overall health and well-being. Incorporating cucumbers into meals and snacks can help increase hydration, provide dietary fiber, and supply vitamins and minerals that are important for various bodily functions.

3.2 Role in a Balanced Diet

Cucumbers play a significant role in promoting a balanced and nutritious diet, offering a range of health benefits while contributing to overall dietary diversity and enjoyment. Here's how cucumbers fit into a balanced diet and why they are an essential component of healthy eating:

1. **Hydration and Refreshment:**

- Cucumbers are primarily composed of water, with a high water content of approximately 95% to 96%. Consuming cucumbers can help maintain hydration levels, especially during hot weather or after physical activity. Their refreshing and hydrating properties make them an excellent choice for staying cool and replenishing fluids.

2. **Low in Calories and Fat:**

- Cucumbers are naturally low in calories and fat, making them a great option for individuals looking to manage their weight or reduce calorie intake. Incorporating cucumbers into meals and snacks can help increase satiety and promote feelings of fullness without adding excess calories or fat.

3. **Rich in Nutrients and Antioxidants:**

- Despite their low calorie and fat content, cucumbers are packed with essential nutrients, vitamins, and antioxidants that contribute to overall health and well-being. They provide a range of vitamins, including vitamin K, vitamin C, and vitamin A, as well as minerals such as potassium and magnesium. These nutrients support various bodily functions, including immune function, bone health, and cardiovascular health.

4. **Dietary Fiber for Digestive Health:**

- Cucumbers are a good source of dietary fiber, with approximately 0.5 to 1 gram of fiber per 100 grams serving. Fiber is essential for digestive health, promoting regular bowel movements, preventing constipation, and supporting gut microbiome diversity. Including cucumbers in meals and snacks can help increase fiber intake and promote overall digestive well-being.

5. **Versatility and Culinary Appeal:**

- Cucumbers are incredibly versatile and can be enjoyed in a variety of ways, from fresh salads and sandwiches to pickles, soups, and smoothies. Their mild flavor and crisp texture make them a versatile ingredient that complements a wide range of dishes and cuisines. Experimenting with different cucumber varieties and culinary techniques can add excitement and variety to meals while increasing overall nutrient intake.

6. **Promotion of Vegetable Consumption:**

- Incorporating cucumbers into meals and snacks can help promote vegetable consumption and increase overall dietary diversity. Including a variety of colorful vegetables, such as cucumbers, in the diet provides a wide range of vitamins, minerals, and phytonutrients that support optimal health and vitality.

7. **Support for Weight Management and Healthy Eating Habits:**

- Cucumbers can play a role in weight management and healthy eating habits by providing a low-calorie, nutrient-dense option for satisfying hunger and cravings. Snacking on cucumbers instead of calorie-dense, processed foods can help reduce overall calorie intake while increasing nutrient intake and promoting satiety.

cucumbers are a valuable addition to a balanced diet, offering hydration, essential nutrients, dietary fiber, and culinary versatility. Including cucumbers in meals and snacks can help promote overall health and well-being while supporting weight management, digestive health, and healthy eating habits. Whether enjoyed fresh, pickled, or incorporated into dishes, cucumbers contribute to a diverse and nutritious diet that nourishes the body and delights the palate.

3.3 Health Benefits and Potential Risks

Cucumbers offer a range of health benefits due to their nutrient-rich composition, high water content, and antioxidant properties. However, like any food, they may also pose potential risks under certain circumstances.

Here's a balanced overview of the health benefits and potential risks associated with consuming cucumbers:

Health Benefits:

1. **Hydration and Nutrient Intake:**

   - Cucumbers are composed primarily of water, making them an excellent hydrating food. Adequate hydration is essential for various bodily functions, including temperature regulation, digestion, and nutrient transport. Consuming cucumbers can help maintain hydration levels, especially during hot weather or after physical activity.

2. **Rich in Vitamins and Minerals:**

   - Cucumbers are a good source of vitamins and minerals, including vitamin K, vitamin C, potassium, and magnesium. These nutrients play vital roles in immune function, bone health, cardiovascular health, and muscle function. Including cucumbers in meals and snacks can help increase overall nutrient intake and support optimal health and well-being.

3. **Antioxidant Properties:**

- Cucumbers contain antioxidants such as beta-carotene, vitamin C, and flavonoids, which help neutralize harmful free radicals and reduce oxidative stress in the body. Antioxidants play a crucial role in protecting cells from damage, supporting immune function, and reducing the risk of chronic diseases such as heart disease, cancer, and diabetes.

4. **Digestive Health:**

- Cucumbers are a good source of dietary fiber, which promotes digestive health by supporting regular bowel movements, preventing constipation, and feeding beneficial gut bacteria. Fiber also helps regulate blood sugar levels, reduce cholesterol levels, and promote satiety, which can aid in weight management.

5. **Skin Health and Beauty:**

- Cucumbers contain compounds such as silica and antioxidants that support skin health and hydration. Applying cucumber slices or cucumber-based skincare products topically may help soothe irritated skin, reduce inflammation, and improve overall complexion. Additionally, consuming cucumbers internally can contribute to healthy, glowing skin from the inside out.

Potential Risks:

1. **Pesticide Residues:**

   - Conventionally grown cucumbers may contain pesticide residues, which can pose potential health risks if consumed in large quantities or without proper washing. To minimize exposure to pesticides, choose organic cucumbers whenever possible and wash conventionally grown cucumbers thoroughly before eating.

2. **Oxalates and Allergies:**

   - Cucumbers contain oxalates, naturally occurring compounds that can contribute to kidney stone formation in susceptible individuals. People with a history of kidney stones or

oxalate-related health issues
may need to limit their intake
of high-oxalate foods,
including cucumbers.
Additionally, some
individuals may be allergic to
cucumbers or develop
allergic reactions, such as
itching, swelling, or hives,
upon consumption.

3. **Digestive Discomfort:**

- Consuming large quantities
  of cucumbers, particularly
  with the skin intact, may
  cause digestive discomfort in
  some individuals, such as
  bloating, gas, or indigestion.
  This may be due to the
  presence of insoluble fiber or
  certain compounds in
  cucumbers that can be
  difficult to digest for some
  people. Moderation and
  mindful consumption can
  help minimize the risk of
  digestive issues.

4. **Potential Contaminants:**

- Cucumbers, especially those grown in contaminated soil or water, may be at risk of microbial contamination, including bacteria such as E. coli or Salmonella. To reduce the risk of foodborne illness, wash cucumbers thoroughly before consumption, and store them properly in the refrigerator.

Cucumbers offer numerous health benefits due to their hydrating properties, nutrient content, and antioxidant effects. However, it's essential to be aware of potential risks associated with pesticide residues, oxalates, allergies, digestive discomfort, and microbial contamination. By consuming cucumbers in moderation, choosing organic options when possible, and practicing proper food safety measures, individuals can enjoy the health benefits of cucumbers while minimizing potential risks to their health and well-being.

CHAPTER 4

Culinary Uses of Cucumber

4.1 Culinary Versatility

Cucumbers are incredibly versatile ingredients that can be incorporated into a wide range of culinary creations, from refreshing salads to savory appetizers and even beverages. Their crisp texture, mild flavor, and high-water content make them a favorite in cuisines around the world. Here's a glimpse into the culinary versatility of cucumbers:

1. **Fresh Salads:**

   - Cucumbers are a staple ingredient in fresh salads, adding a crunchy texture and refreshing flavor. They pair well with leafy greens, tomatoes, onions, and herbs, and can be dressed with vinaigrettes, yogurt-based dressings, or citrus-infused marinades.

2. **Sandwiches and Wraps:**

- Sliced cucumbers are a classic addition to sandwiches, wraps, and pitas, providing a crisp contrast to savory fillings such as deli meats, cheeses, hummus, or spreads. They can also be pickled or marinated for added flavor.

3. **Appetizers and Snacks:**

- Cucumbers make excellent appetizers and snacks when served raw or lightly seasoned. Cucumber slices can be topped with cream cheese, smoked salmon, or tzatziki sauce for elegant hors d'oeuvres. Alternatively, cucumber sticks or spears can be served with dips, such as hummus, guacamole, or ranch dressing, for a refreshing snack.

4. **Pickles and Fermented Foods:**

- Cucumbers are perhaps best known for their role in pickling, a preservation technique that imparts tangy, savory flavors to the crisp cucumbers. Pickled cucumbers, or "pickles," can be sweet, sour, spicy, or dill-flavored, depending on the pickling method and seasoning used. Additionally, cucumbers can be fermented to create probiotic-rich foods such as kimchi or sauerkraut.

5. **Soups and Gazpachos:**

- Cucumbers add a refreshing element to cold soups and gazpachos, blending well with ingredients such as tomatoes, bell peppers, onions, and herbs. Chilled cucumber soup, often seasoned with yogurt, dill, or mint, is a popular summertime dish in many cultures.

6. **Beverages and Infusions:**

   - Cucumbers can be used to infuse flavor into water, lemonade, or cocktails, adding a subtle, cooling essence to beverages. Cucumber-infused water is a popular choice for hydration, while cucumber-based cocktails, such as the classic "cucumber cooler," are refreshing options for warm weather.

7. **Sushi and Rolls:**

   - Cucumber slices or sticks are a common ingredient in sushi and sushi rolls, providing a crunchy texture and mild flavor that balances the richness of fish, rice, and nori seaweed. Cucumber rolls, or "kappa maki," are a vegetarian sushi option that highlights the simplicity and versatility of cucumbers.

8. **Sauces and Dips:**

- Cucumbers can be pureed or finely chopped to create sauces, dips, and condiments with a fresh, vibrant taste. Tzatziki, a Greek yogurt and cucumber sauce flavored with garlic and dill, is a popular accompaniment to grilled meats, kebabs, and gyros. Cucumber salsa, made with diced cucumbers, tomatoes, onions, and jalapenos, adds a refreshing twist to Mexican-inspired dishes.

9. **Side Dishes and Accompaniments:**

- Cucumbers can be served as a simple side dish or accompaniment to main courses, providing a light and refreshing contrast to richer flavors. Cucumber salads, marinated cucumbers, or cucumber relishes are common side dishes in various cuisines, offering a burst of freshness and texture to the meal.

cucumbers offer endless culinary possibilities, from salads and sandwiches to pickles, soups, beverages, and beyond. Their versatility, mild flavor, and crisp texture make them a favorite ingredient in kitchens worldwide, where they add freshness, hydration, and a burst of flavor to a wide range of dishes and culinary creations. Whether enjoyed raw, pickled, or cooked, cucumbers are sure to delight the palate and enhance the dining experience in countless ways.

4.2 Traditional and Contemporary Recipes

Cucumbers are a versatile ingredient that can be used in a variety of traditional and contemporary recipes, ranging from classic salads to innovative dishes that showcase their flavor and texture. Here are examples of both traditional and contemporary cucumber recipes:

Traditional Recipes:

1. **Greek Tzatziki:**

   - Tzatziki is a classic Greek dip or sauce made with strained yogurt, grated cucumber, garlic, lemon juice, and fresh herbs such as dill or mint. It is often served as a condiment with grilled meats, gyros, or as a dip for pita bread and vegetables.

2. **Japanese Sunomono Salad:**

   - Sunomono is a traditional Japanese cucumber salad

made with thinly sliced
cucumbers, rice vinegar,
sugar, and soy sauce. It is
often garnished with sesame
seeds, seaweed, or thinly
sliced ginger and served as a
refreshing side dish or
appetizer.

3. **Indian Cucumber Raita:**

    - Raita is a traditional Indian
      yogurt-based condiment
      flavored with grated
      cucumber, cumin, coriander,
      and mint. It is typically
      served alongside spicy
      curries, biryanis, or grilled
      meats to cool the palate and
      complement the richness of
      the main dish.

4. **Russian Cucumber Salad (Salat
    Ogurets):**

    - Russian cucumber salad, or
      salat ogurets, is a simple
      salad made with thinly sliced

cucumbers, onions, dill, sour cream, and vinegar. It is a popular side dish served alongside hearty Russian meals, such as stews, soups, or dumplings.

5. **Middle Eastern Fattoush Salad:**

- Fattoush is a traditional Middle Eastern salad made with a combination of cucumbers, tomatoes, lettuce, radishes, and herbs, such as parsley and mint. It is typically dressed with a tangy sumac and lemon vinaigrette and topped with crispy pieces of toasted pita bread.

Contemporary Recipes:

1. **Cucumber and Avocado Sushi Rolls:**

- Contemporary sushi rolls featuring cucumber and avocado are a popular vegetarian option that showcases the crisp texture and mild flavor of cucumbers. Rolled with sushi rice and nori seaweed, these sushi rolls are a refreshing and satisfying meal or appetizer.

2. **Cucumber Noodle Salad with Peanut Sauce:**

   - Cucumber noodle salad is a contemporary twist on traditional salads, featuring spiralized cucumbers as the base instead of traditional greens. Tossed with a creamy peanut sauce, shredded carrots, bell peppers, and fresh herbs, this salad is light, flavorful, and satisfying.

3. **Cucumber Mint Gazpacho:**

   - Gazpacho is a chilled Spanish soup traditionally made with tomatoes, peppers, onions, and cucumbers. A contemporary variation of gazpacho incorporates cucumbers and mint for a refreshing twist on this classic dish. Blended with yogurt or coconut milk for creaminess, cucumber mint gazpacho is a perfect summer appetizer or light meal.

4. **Grilled Cucumber and Halloumi Skewers:**

- Grilled cucumber and halloumi skewers are a contemporary take on traditional kebabs, featuring marinated cucumber slices and cubes of halloumi cheese threaded onto skewers and grilled until golden and caramelized. Served with a tangy yogurt sauce or salsa verde, these skewers make a delicious appetizer or main course.

5. **Cucumber Watermelon Salad with Feta and Mint:**

- A contemporary salad that combines sweet watermelon, salty feta cheese, and crisp cucumbers, all tossed with fresh mint and a tangy vinaigrette. This vibrant and refreshing salad is a celebration of summer flavors and textures.

cucumbers lend themselves to a wide range of traditional and contemporary recipes, from classic salads and dips to innovative dishes that showcase their versatility and flavor. Whether enjoyed in traditional dishes from around the world or incorporated into contemporary creations, cucumbers add freshness, texture, and a burst of flavor to any meal.

4.3 Preservation and Storage Techniques

Preserving and storing cucumbers properly is essential to maintain their freshness, flavor, and nutritional value. Whether you have an abundance of cucumbers from your garden or want to prolong their shelf life from the grocery store, here are some effective preservation and storage techniques:

1. **Refrigeration:**

   - The most common method for storing cucumbers is refrigeration. Place whole, unwashed cucumbers in the vegetable crisper drawer of your refrigerator. They should be kept away from ethylene-producing fruits like apples and bananas, as exposure to ethylene can accelerate spoilage.

   - Cucumbers stored in the refrigerator can last up to one

to two weeks, depending on
their freshness at the time of
purchase or harvest.

2. **Wrapping:**

- To extend the shelf life of
  cucumbers, wrap them
  individually in paper towels
  before refrigerating. This
  helps absorb excess moisture
  and prevents them from
  becoming soggy, which can
  lead to spoilage.

- Alternatively, you can store
  cucumbers in perforated
  plastic bags or reusable
  produce bags designed for
  storing fresh produce. These
  bags allow for proper airflow
  while retaining moisture,
  keeping the cucumbers crisp
  and fresh for longer.

3. **Pickling:**

- Pickling is a popular
  preservation method that

enhances the flavor and texture of cucumbers while extending their shelf life. To pickle cucumbers, slice or spear them and pack them tightly into sterilized jars with brine made from vinegar, water, salt, sugar, and spices.

- Process the jars in a boiling water bath canner according to a tested recipe to ensure safe preservation. Pickled cucumbers, also known as pickles, can be stored in a cool, dark place for up to one year.

4. **Freezing:**

- While cucumbers are not typically frozen for long-term storage due to their high-water content, they can be frozen for use in certain dishes such as smoothies or soups. To freeze cucumbers, slice or chop them and blanch them in boiling water for 1-2 minutes.

- Transfer the blanched cucumbers to an ice water bath to stop the cooking process, then drain and pat them dry. Place the cucumbers in a single layer on a baking sheet and freeze until solid before transferring them to freezer-safe containers or bags for long-term storage in the freezer.

5. **Dehydrating:**

- Dehydrating cucumbers is another preservation method that removes moisture from the cucumbers, resulting in a crispy texture similar to chips. To dehydrate cucumbers, slice them thinly and arrange them in a single layer on a dehydrator tray.

- Dry the cucumbers at a low temperature (around 125°F to 135°F or 52°C to 57°C) until they are crisp and brittle. Store the dehydrated cucumbers in an airtight container in a cool, dry place for up to several months.

6. **Fermentation:**

- Fermenting cucumbers is a traditional preservation method that results in tangy, probiotic-rich pickles. To ferment cucumbers, submerge them in a brine solution made from salt and water in a fermentation vessel such as a crock or jar.

- Allow the cucumbers to ferment at room temperature for several days to several weeks, depending on your preference for taste and texture. Once fermented, store the pickles in the refrigerator to slow down the fermentation process and preserve their flavor and texture.

Utilizing these preservation and storage techniques, you can enjoy fresh cucumbers throughout the year and minimize food waste while adding flavor and nutrition to your meals. Whether you prefer crisp, raw cucumbers in salads and sandwiches or tangy, preserved cucumbers in pickles and relishes, there are plenty of options to suit your taste preferences and culinary needs.

CHAPTER 5

Economic Importance and Commercial Applications

5.1 Global Production and Market Trends

Cucumbers hold significant economic importance worldwide, both as a widely consumed vegetable and as a key agricultural commodity. Understanding global production and market trends provides insights into the economic significance and commercial applications of cucumbers. Here's an overview of global cucumber production and market trends:

1. **Production Trends:**

    - Cucumbers are cultivated in various regions around the world, with production

concentrated in both
temperate and tropical
climates. Major cucumber-
producing countries include
China, Turkey, Russia, Iran,
and the United States.

- China is the largest producer
  of cucumbers globally,
  accounting for a significant
  portion of total production.
  The country's vast
  agricultural land, favorable
  growing conditions, and
  advanced cultivation
  techniques contribute to its
  dominance in the cucumber
  market.

- Other top cucumber-
  producing countries often
  vary depending on factors
  such as climate, agricultural
  practices, and market
  demand. In regions with
  favorable growing
  conditions, cucumbers are
  cultivated year-round, while

in temperate climates,
production may be seasonal.

2. **Market Trends:**

- The global cucumber market
  is influenced by factors such
  as population growth,
  consumer preferences,
  dietary habits, and economic
  conditions. Cucumbers are
  consumed fresh, pickled, or
  processed into various food
  products, catering to diverse
  culinary preferences and
  cultural traditions.

- The demand for cucumbers
  continues to grow steadily
  due to increasing awareness
  of their nutritional benefits,
  versatility in culinary
  applications, and popularity
  in global cuisines.
  Cucumbers are valued for
  their crisp texture, mild
  flavor, and high water
  content, making them a

favorite ingredient in salads, sandwiches, snacks, and pickles.

- In addition to fresh consumption, cucumbers are used in commercial food processing industries to produce pickles, relishes, sauces, soups, and beverages. Processed cucumber products offer convenience, extended shelf life, and value-added options for consumers seeking ready-to-eat or convenience foods.

- Market trends also reflect shifts in consumer preferences towards healthier, natural, and organic food choices. Organic cucumbers, grown without synthetic pesticides or fertilizers, are increasingly sought after by health-conscious consumers concerned about food safety,

environmental sustainability,
and ethical farming practices.

3. **Export and Import Dynamics:**

- Cucumber trade occurs
  between countries to meet
  domestic demand, fill
  seasonal gaps, and take
  advantage of price
  differentials. Major
  cucumber-exporting
  countries supply fresh
  cucumbers, pickles, and
  processed cucumber products
  to international markets,
  while importing countries
  rely on imports to supplement
  domestic production or meet
  specific market demands.

- Trade agreements, tariffs,
  transportation costs, and
  quality standards influence
  the dynamics of cucumber
  trade between countries.
  Export-oriented economies
  often invest in infrastructure,

logistics, and quality control measures to maintain competitiveness in the global market and ensure product traceability and safety.

- Cucumber trade is also influenced by regional preferences, culinary traditions, and cultural factors. For example, pickled cucumbers, a staple in some cuisines, may have higher demand in regions where pickling is a traditional preservation method or where pickled products are valued as condiments or snacks.

Global cucumber production and market trends reflect the economic importance and commercial applications of cucumbers as a versatile and widely consumed vegetable. Understanding production dynamics, market trends, and trade patterns provides valuable insights for stakeholders in the agricultural, food processing, and retail sectors, enabling informed decision-making, strategic planning, and market positioning within the global cucumber industry.

5.2 Industrial Uses and Processing

Cucumbers have numerous industrial applications beyond their role as a fresh vegetable. From processing into pickles to extraction for cosmetic and pharmaceutical purposes, cucumbers offer diverse opportunities for commercial utilization. Here's an overview of some industrial uses and processing techniques:

1. **Pickling:**

    - One of the most common industrial uses of cucumbers is for pickling. Cucumbers are processed into pickles through fermentation or vinegar brining methods. The pickling industry produces various types of pickles, including dill pickles, bread and butter pickles, sweet pickles, and gherkins, to cater to different taste preferences and market demands.

2. **Cucumber Extracts in Cosmetics:**

    - Cucumber extracts are valued in the cosmetics industry for their soothing, hydrating, and anti-inflammatory properties. Cucumber extracts are incorporated into skincare products such as moisturizers, toners, serums, and eye creams to provide hydration, reduce redness and puffiness, and promote skin health.

3. **Cucumber Extracts in Pharmaceuticals:**

    - Cucumber extracts are also utilized in pharmaceutical formulations for their potential health benefits. Cucumber extract supplements or dietary supplements may be marketed for their antioxidant properties, anti-inflammatory effects, and potential to support skin health, digestion, and overall well-being.

4. **Cucumber Juice and Concentrates:**

- Cucumbers can be processed into juice and concentrates for use in beverages, food products, and culinary applications. Cucumber juice and concentrates may be used as a base for smoothies, cocktails, and flavored water, or incorporated into sauces, soups, and salad dressings for added flavor and nutrition.

5. **Cucumber Powder and Flakes:**

- Cucumber powder and flakes are produced by dehydrating

cucumbers and grinding them into a fine powder or flakes. Cucumber powder and flakes can be used as flavoring agents, seasoning blends, or nutritional supplements in food products, snacks, and supplements. They may also be used as natural colorants or additives in cosmetic and pharmaceutical formulations.

6. **Cucumber Seed Oil:**

- Cucumber seed oil is extracted from cucumber seeds and valued for its moisturizing, emollient, and antioxidant properties. Cucumber seed oil is used in skincare products such as moisturizers, lotions, and facial oils to hydrate and nourish the skin, reduce inflammation, and protect against environmental damage.

7. **Cucumber Fiber:**

- Cucumber fiber is a byproduct of cucumber processing that can be used as a dietary fiber supplement or functional ingredient in food products. Cucumber fiber may be incorporated into baked goods, cereals, snack bars, and other food products to increase fiber content, improve texture, and enhance nutritional value.

8. **Cucumber Vinegar:**

- Cucumber vinegar is a type of vinegar made from fermented cucumber juice or cucumber slices. Cucumber vinegar may be used as a salad dressing, marinade, or flavoring agent in culinary applications. It may also have potential uses in pickling, food preservation, and traditional medicine.

9. **Cucumber Extracts in Personal Care Products:**

- Cucumber extracts are commonly used in personal care products such as shampoos, conditioners, and body washes for their refreshing scent and moisturizing properties. Cucumber extracts may also be found in bath products, perfumes, and aromatherapy formulations for their uplifting and invigorating aroma.

cucumbers have diverse industrial uses and processing applications, ranging from pickling to extraction for cosmetic, pharmaceutical, and food applications. The versatility of cucumbers as a raw material offers opportunities for innovation and product development in various industries, contributing to their economic importance and commercial value beyond their role as a fresh vegetable.

5.3 Trade and Economic Impact

The trade of cucumbers and cucumber-derived products has a significant economic impact globally, affecting agricultural sectors, food industries, and international commerce. Understanding the trade dynamics and economic implications of cucumbers provides insights into their value chain and contribution to global economies. Here's an overview of the trade and economic impact of cucumbers:

1. **Export and Import Markets:**

   - Cucumbers are traded internationally to meet domestic demand, fill seasonal gaps, and take advantage of comparative advantages in production. Major cucumber-exporting countries, such as China, Turkey, Iran, Russia, and the United States, supply fresh cucumbers, pickles, and processed cucumber products to global markets.

- Importing countries rely on cucumber imports to supplement domestic production, cater to specific market demands, and maintain year-round availability. Importers may source cucumbers from multiple countries based on factors such as price, quality, freshness, and proximity to markets.

2. **Trade Agreements and Tariffs:**

- Trade agreements, tariffs, and non-tariff barriers influence the flow of cucumbers and cucumber-derived products between countries. Bilateral and multilateral trade agreements may facilitate or restrict cucumber trade by reducing tariffs, harmonizing standards, and streamlining customs procedures.

- Tariffs and import duties imposed on cucumbers can affect the competitiveness of exporting countries and the affordability of cucumbers for consumers in importing countries. Trade negotiations and diplomatic efforts may seek to address trade barriers and promote fair and transparent trade practices.

3. **Economic Value Chain:**

- The cucumber value chain encompasses various stages of production, processing, distribution, and consumption, generating economic value and employment opportunities along the way. Cucumber cultivation involves farmers, laborers, and agricultural

inputs such as seeds,
fertilizers, and machinery.

- Processing industries add
  value to cucumbers by
  producing pickles, sauces,
  juices, extracts, and other
  value-added products. These
  processed cucumber products
  contribute to the food
  processing sector's output,
  employment, and revenue
  generation.

- Trade and distribution
  channels, including
  wholesalers, retailers, and
  exporters, play a crucial role
  in connecting producers with
  consumers and facilitating
  the flow of cucumbers and
  cucumber products in
  domestic and international
  markets.

4. **Economic Impact on Producers
   and Consumers:**

- Cucumber trade can have both positive and negative economic impacts on producers and consumers. Export-oriented cucumber producers may benefit from access to global markets, increased demand, and higher prices for their products. However, they may also face challenges such as price volatility, competition, and market access barriers.

- Importing countries may benefit from access to a diverse range of cucumbers and cucumber products, ensuring year-round availability and satisfying consumer preferences. However, they may also face challenges such as import dependency, trade imbalances, and food safety concerns.

- Consumers in importing countries may benefit from access to affordable cucumbers and cucumber products, enhancing dietary diversity, nutrition, and culinary experiences. However, they may also be exposed to quality issues, price fluctuations, and supply chain disruptions.

5. **Market Trends and Opportunities:**

- Market trends, consumer preferences, and technological advancements drive innovation and opportunities in the cucumber trade. Growing demand for fresh, organic, and minimally processed cucumbers reflects changing consumer lifestyles, health consciousness, and culinary trends.

- Opportunities for value addition, product

differentiation, and market segmentation exist in the cucumber trade, including premium varieties, organic certifications, convenience packaging, and functional ingredients. Investment in research and development, marketing strategies, and supply chain logistics can enhance competitiveness and market access for cucumber producers and exporters.

Cucumber trade and its economic impact are influenced by factors such as trade agreements, tariffs, value chain dynamics, consumer preferences, and market trends. Understanding these factors helps stakeholders navigate opportunities and challenges in the global cucumber trade, contributing to sustainable growth, economic development, and food security across regions.

CHAPTER 6

Future Prospects and Research Directions

6.1 Emerging Trends in Cucumber Production

Cucumber production is evolving to meet the demands of changing consumer preferences, technological advancements, and environmental sustainability. Emerging trends in cucumber production reflect efforts to optimize yields, enhance quality, and minimize environmental impact. Here are some key emerging trends in cucumber production:

1. **Vertical Farming and Controlled Environment Agriculture:**

   - Vertical farming and controlled environment agriculture (CEA) methods are gaining traction in cucumber production. These innovative techniques involve growing cucumbers in vertically stacked layers or indoor facilities equipped with artificial lighting, climate control, and hydroponic or aeroponic systems.

- Vertical farming and CEA offer advantages such as year-round production, higher yields per square meter, reduced water usage, and protection against pests and diseases. These methods also enable growers to optimize resource utilization, minimize environmental footprint, and produce cucumbers closer to urban markets.

2. **Hydroponic and Aeroponic Systems:**

- Hydroponic and aeroponic systems are increasingly used in cucumber production to grow plants without soil, using nutrient-rich water or misted air instead. These soilless cultivation methods offer precise control over nutrient delivery, water management, and plant growth parameters.

- Hydroponic and aeroponic cucumber production systems can be integrated into vertical farms, greenhouses, or urban agriculture initiatives, enabling year-round production in diverse environments. These systems promote resource efficiency, minimize pesticide use, and enhance crop quality and consistency.

3. **Protected Cultivation and High-Tech Greenhouses:**

- Protected cultivation techniques, such as greenhouse farming, are evolving with the adoption of high-tech solutions and smart technologies. Modern greenhouses are equipped with automated climate control systems, sensors, irrigation management, and data analytics tools to optimize growing conditions and maximize productivity.

- High-tech greenhouses provide cucumbers with ideal growing conditions, including temperature, humidity, light intensity, and carbon dioxide levels, leading to higher yields, superior quality, and extended growing seasons. These advanced facilities also enable growers to mitigate climate risks, reduce resource consumption, and improve crop resilience.

4. **Precision Agriculture and Digital Farming:**

- Precision agriculture and digital farming technologies are transforming cucumber production by enabling data-driven decision-making, real-time monitoring, and targeted interventions. These technologies include satellite imagery, drones, GPS-guided machinery, and sensor networks for soil and crop monitoring.

- Precision agriculture tools allow cucumber growers to optimize inputs such as water, fertilizers, and pesticides, reducing waste and environmental impact. By adopting data-driven approaches, growers can improve crop health, yield predictability, and resource efficiency, leading to more sustainable and profitable cucumber production.

5. **Biological Control and Integrated Pest Management (IPM):**

- Biological control methods and integrated pest management (IPM) strategies are gaining importance in cucumber production as alternatives to chemical pesticides. Biological control agents, such as predatory insects, parasitic nematodes, and microbial biopesticides, help manage pests while minimizing environmental harm.

- Integrated pest management combines biological, cultural, and chemical control tactics to prevent pest outbreaks, reduce pesticide reliance, and preserve natural ecosystems.

By promoting biodiversity, enhancing soil health, and minimizing chemical residues, IPM contributes to sustainable cucumber production and food safety.

6. **Genetic Improvement and Breeding Programs:**

- Genetic improvement and breeding programs aim to develop cucumber varieties with enhanced traits such as disease resistance, tolerance to abiotic stress, improved yield potential, and superior quality attributes. Advances in genomics, molecular breeding, and gene editing technologies accelerate the breeding process and expand the genetic diversity available to breeders.

- Breeding programs focus on consumer-preferred traits such as flavor, texture, color, and shelf life, as well as traits related to sustainability, such as water use efficiency, heat tolerance, and resistance to emerging pests and diseases. By harnessing genetic diversity and cutting-edge breeding tools, breeders can develop cucumbers that meet the evolving needs of growers, processors, retailers, and consumers.

Emerging trends in cucumber production reflect efforts to enhance efficiency, sustainability, and resilience in response to evolving market demands and environmental challenges. By embracing innovation, adopting advanced technologies, and integrating holistic approaches, cucumber producers can optimize productivity, improve quality, and contribute to a more sustainable and resilient food system. Ongoing research and collaboration across disciplines will continue to drive innovation and shape the future of cucumber production in a rapidly changing agricultural landscape.

6.2 Innovations in Genetics and Biotechnology

Advancements in genetics and biotechnology have revolutionized cucumber breeding, crop improvement, and agricultural sustainability. These innovations offer new tools and techniques for addressing challenges such as pest resistance, disease management, climate resilience, and nutritional quality. Here are some key innovations in genetics and biotechnology shaping the future of cucumber production:

1. **Genomic Sequencing and Marker-Assisted Breeding:**

    - Genomic sequencing of cucumber genomes has provided valuable insights into the genetic basis of important traits such as disease resistance, fruit quality, and stress tolerance. Marker-assisted breeding techniques leverage genomic information to accelerate the breeding process by identifying and selecting plants with desired traits at the molecular level.

- Marker-assisted breeding enables breeders to develop cucumber varieties with improved traits more efficiently and precisely, leading to faster and more targeted crop improvement. By combining traditional breeding methods with molecular tools, breeders can introgress valuable traits from wild relatives or exotic germplasm into cultivated varieties, enhancing genetic diversity and resilience.

2. **Gene Editing Technologies:**

- Gene editing technologies, such as CRISPR-Cas9, offer precise and targeted methods for modifying the cucumber genome to introduce or enhance desirable traits. CRISPR-Cas9 allows researchers to edit specific genes involved in traits such as disease resistance, fruit size, color, and nutritional content.

- Gene editing accelerates the breeding process by enabling precise modifications without introducing foreign DNA, thus avoiding regulatory hurdles associated with genetically modified organisms (GMOs). By harnessing gene editing technologies, breeders can develop cucumber varieties with enhanced traits while maintaining genetic purity and consumer acceptance.

3. **Transgenic Approaches for Trait Introduction:**

- Transgenic approaches involve the introduction of foreign genes into the cucumber genome to confer desired traits such as insect resistance, herbicide tolerance, or abiotic stress tolerance. Transgenic cucumbers have been developed with traits such as resistance to cucumber mosaic virus (CMV), powdery mildew, or insect pests.

- Transgenic cucumbers offer potential solutions to challenges such as pest and disease management, particularly in regions where conventional breeding methods have limitations. However, regulatory approval, public acceptance, and market access may pose challenges for the commercialization of transgenic cucumbers in some countries or markets.

4. **Omics Technologies for Trait Discovery:**

- Omics technologies, including genomics, transcriptomics, proteomics, and metabolomics, enable comprehensive analysis of the cucumber genome, gene expression, protein composition, and metabolite profiles. These high-throughput techniques facilitate trait discovery, functional characterization, and molecular breeding.

- Omics approaches provide insights into the complex genetic and biochemical networks underlying important traits in cucumbers, such as fruit development, stress responses, and nutritional quality. By integrating omics data with phenotypic information, researchers can identify candidate genes and metabolic pathways for targeted crop improvement.

5. **Bioinformatics and Computational Biology:**

- Bioinformatics and computational biology play critical roles in analyzing and interpreting large-scale genomic and omics data sets generated from cucumber research. Computational tools and algorithms enable researchers to predict gene functions, identify genetic markers, and model complex biological processes.

- Bioinformatics resources such as genome databases, genetic maps, and gene annotation tools support cucumber breeding programs, trait discovery, and molecular breeding efforts. By leveraging computational approaches, researchers can accelerate the pace of genetic discovery and crop improvement in cucumbers.

6. **Synthetic Biology and Metabolic Engineering:**

   - Synthetic biology and metabolic engineering approaches aim to engineer metabolic pathways in cucumbers to enhance desirable traits such as nutritional quality, flavor, aroma, and shelf life. These techniques involve manipulating enzyme activities, pathway fluxes, and metabolite profiles to optimize fruit characteristics.

- Synthetic biology strategies may involve the introduction of genes from other organisms or the modification of endogenous metabolic pathways to produce desired compounds or enhance metabolic efficiency. By reprogramming metabolic networks, researchers can create cucumbers with improved sensory attributes, nutritional profiles, and postharvest qualities.

Innovations in genetics and biotechnology are revolutionizing cucumber breeding, crop improvement, and agricultural sustainability. These advancements offer new tools and strategies for enhancing traits such as disease resistance, stress tolerance, nutritional quality, and market appeal. By leveraging cutting-edge technologies and interdisciplinary approaches, researchers and breeders can develop cucumbers that meet the evolving needs of growers, processors, retailers, and consumers in a rapidly changing agricultural landscape. Ongoing collaboration, regulatory oversight, and public engagement will be essential to ensure the responsible and beneficial use of genetic and biotechnological innovations in cucumber production.

6.3 Sustainability and Environmental Considerations

As cucumber production continues to expand to meet global demand, sustainability and environmental considerations are becoming increasingly important. Sustainable practices aim to minimize environmental impact, conserve natural resources, promote biodiversity, and support the long-term viability of cucumber farming systems. Here are key sustainability and environmental considerations in cucumber production:

1. **Water Management:**

- Water is a critical resource in cucumber production, and efficient water management practices are essential for sustainability. Drip irrigation, micro-irrigation, and precision irrigation technologies can optimize water use by delivering water directly to the roots with minimal waste.

- Water recycling and reuse systems can capture and treat irrigation runoff, reducing water consumption and minimizing nutrient leaching. Rainwater harvesting techniques can also supplement irrigation water during dry periods, enhancing water resilience and reducing reliance on groundwater.

2. **Soil Health and Conservation:**

   - Maintaining soil health is vital for sustainable

cucumber production, as
healthy soils support plant
growth, nutrient cycling, and
water infiltration.
Conservation tillage, cover
cropping, and crop rotation
practices can improve soil
structure, reduce erosion, and
enhance soil organic matter
content.

- Integrated soil fertility
  management strategies, such
  as organic amendments,
  green manures, and balanced
  fertilization, promote nutrient
  cycling and minimize
  nutrient losses to the
  environment. Soil testing and
  nutrient management plans
  help optimize fertilizer
  application rates and timing,
  reducing environmental
  pollution and nutrient runoff.

3. **Pest and Disease Management:**

- Integrated pest management (IPM) approaches aim to minimize pesticide use and mitigate environmental risks while effectively managing pests and diseases in cucumber crops. Biological control agents, cultural practices, and resistant varieties can reduce reliance on synthetic pesticides and preserve natural enemies.

- Crop monitoring, scouting, and early detection techniques enable growers to implement timely interventions and prevent pest outbreaks. Adoption of pest-resistant varieties, pheromone traps, and biopesticides can help maintain pest populations below economic thresholds while minimizing environmental impact.

4. **Biodiversity Conservation:**

- Biodiversity conservation measures enhance ecosystem resilience and promote natural pest control in cucumber agroecosystems. Hedgerows, field margins, and wildlife corridors provide habitat for beneficial insects, birds, and other organisms that contribute to pest suppression and pollination.

- Agroforestry systems, agroecological landscapes, and diversified cropping systems integrate trees, shrubs, and multiple crops to enhance biodiversity, soil fertility, and ecosystem services. By mimicking natural ecosystems, these practices support biodiversity conservation and ecological balance in cucumber production areas.

5. **Energy Efficiency and Renewable Energy:**

- Improving energy efficiency and transitioning to renewable energy sources can reduce greenhouse gas emissions and mitigate climate change impacts associated with cucumber production. Energy-efficient technologies such as LED lighting, energy-efficient greenhouse designs, and solar-powered irrigation systems can reduce energy consumption and operating costs.

- On-farm renewable energy systems, such as solar panels, wind turbines, and biogas digesters, can generate clean energy and reduce reliance on fossil fuels. By harnessing renewable energy sources, cucumber growers can enhance energy resilience, reduce carbon footprints, and contribute to climate mitigation efforts.

6. **Waste Reduction and Recycling:**

- Minimizing waste generation and promoting recycling and reuse practices are integral to sustainable cucumber production. On-farm composting of crop residues, kitchen scraps, and organic waste can produce nutrient-rich compost for soil amendment and fertility enhancement.

- Packaging optimization, waste segregation, and recycling programs can reduce packaging waste and promote the use of biodegradable or recyclable materials. Closed-loop systems for water, nutrients, and organic matter management can minimize waste generation and resource losses in cucumber production systems.

7. **Sustainable Supply Chains and Market Access:**

- Promoting sustainable supply chains and market access for sustainably produced cucumbers can incentivize growers to adopt environmentally friendly practices and meet consumer demand for responsibly sourced products. Certification programs, eco-labeling schemes, and fair-trade initiatives can help differentiate sustainably produced cucumbers in the marketplace.

- Collaborative partnerships along the cucumber value chain, including growers, processors, retailers, and consumers, can foster transparency, traceability, and accountability for sustainable production practices. By aligning market incentives with environmental stewardship, stakeholders can support the transition to more sustainable cucumber production systems.

sustainability and environmental considerations are integral to the future of cucumber production, encompassing water management, soil health, pest and disease management, biodiversity conservation, energy efficiency, waste reduction, and sustainable supply chains. By adopting holistic and integrated approaches, cucumber growers can enhance environmental stewardship, promote resilience, and ensure the long-term viability of cucumber farming systems in a changing climate and globalized economy.